Psycholog

Migrai
her Comm

ished in 1926, as
nis title is based
lon Clinical Society
ollege respectively.
idemiologist, and
an be read and enj

Migraine and Other Common Neuroses

A psychological study

F.G. Crookshank

Routledge
Taylor & Francis Group
LONDON AND NEW YORK

First published in 1926
by Kegan Paul, Trench, Trubner & Co. Ltd

This edition first published in 2016 by Routledge
27 Church Road, Hove BN3 2FA

and by Routledge
711 Third Avenue, New York, NY 10017

Routledge is an imprint of the Taylor & Francis Group, an informa business

Publisher's Note

The publisher has gone to great lengths to ensure the quality of this reprint but points out that some imperfections in the original copies may be apparent.

Disclaimer

The publisher has made every effort to trace copyright holders and welcomes correspondence from those they have been unable to contact.

ISBN: 978-1-138-12312-0 (hbk)
ISBN: 978-1-315-64902-3 (ebk)

PSYCHE MINIATURES
Medical Series No. 1

MIGRAINE
AND OTHER COMMON NEUROSES

"*Socrates*, in *Plato*, would prescribe no Physick for *Charmides*' headache *till first he had eased his troublesome mind*; *body and soul must be cured together, as head and eyes.*"

BURTON, *Anatomy of Melancholy*.

PSYCHE MINIATURES

MEDICAL SERIES

Migraine, and other Common Neuroses
by F. G. CROOKSHANK, M.D., F.R.C.P,

Aphasia
by S. A. KINNIER WILSON, M.D., F.R.C.P. (In preparation).

The Morbid Conscience
by PROFESSOR C. BLONDEL, (In preparation).

Types of Mind and Body
by E. MILLER, M.A. (In preparation).

GENERAL

Science and Poetry
by I. A. RICHARDS, M.A. (In the press).

Economics, Ethics and Psychology,
by P. SARGANT FLORENCE, M.A., Ph.D. (In preparation)

The Mind of a Chimpanzee
by C. K. OGDEN. (In preparation).

PUBLISHED IN CONNECTION WITH
" PSYCHE "
A QUARTERLY JOURNAL OF GENERAL AND APPLIED PSYCHOLGY

MIGRAINE
and Other Common Neuroses

A PSYCHOLOGICAL STUDY

BY

F. G. CROOKSHANK, M.D., F.R.C.P.

Physician to the Prince of Wales' General Hospital and to the French Hospital, London

KEGAN PAUL, TRENCH, TRUBNER & CO., LTD.
Broadway House: 68-74 Carter Lane, London, E.C.
1926

By the Same Author

The Mongol in our Midst (*2nd Edn.*), 1925.

Influenza, 1922.

Essays and Clinical Studies, 1911.

Made and Printed in Great Britain by
M. F. Robinson & Co., Ltd., at The Library Press, Lowestoft

NOTE BY THE AUTHOR

These two lectures are here reprinted, with but little alteration in spite of some repetition, in the hope that the interest of practitioners may be drawn towards consideration of the psychical no less than the physical, and the physical no less than the psychical aspect of every case of ' neurosis ' and ' functional ' disease.

Particular attention is paid to the discussion of migraine and allied paroxysmal neuroses, for the facts thereof are easily verifiable by anyone who is not content with simple expressions of incredulity.

But other neuroses — ' colitis ,' asthma of a kind, aerophagia, ' false ' angina pectoris and the like—may each be profitably subjected to analysis, and will be found, in each and every case, to be associated with a psychical state as characteristic and easily recognizable as is that of migraine and trigeminal neuralgia.

For too long, teachers of medicine have insisted upon a false antithesis between so-called "functional" or "neurotic" maladies and those supposed to rest upon an "organic" basis. The unprejudiced physician will find some physical defect in every "functional" case, and some psychical factor in every case of "organic disease."

For permission to reprint, I am indebted to the Editors of *Psyche* and *The Medical Press and Circular* respectively.

F. G. C.

CONTENTS

I

THE PSYCHOLOGICAL INTEREST IN THE COMMON NEUROSES

When, as an Asylum Medical Officer some thirty years ago, I first began to recognize that every person who is ill is ill psychically as well as physically, I hoped and believed that the rectification of disordered psychical states was best brought about by the rectification of the disordered physical states; just as "that Krüschen feeling" is said, and sometimes is, to be brought about by a dose of salts. But, apart from my experience in particular cases, I fear that I accepted this as a principle of general value because at that time I believed in the odd sort of psychophysical parallelism, bred by agnosticism out of materialism, then so

[1] A Lecture given before the North-East London Clinical Society: 1925.

deplorably current. I now believe, as a result of experience and reflection that, though we can often secure psychical amelioration when we treat patients physically, and though we often fail—and must fail, unless we have faith as a grain of mustard seed that will remove mountains and cast them into yonder sea—although we fail, I say, to cure certain physical ailments by what are called pyschical methods: nevertheless, the last word, the final choice, is more often than we think, with ourselves: with our Will. Mind has the casting vote, and is the predominant partner: what we call the body is at some time or another subordinate to it. If I have come to abandon belief in the agnostic psycho-physical parallelism of Herbert Spencer, Huxley, and Hughlings Jackson, I am only one of very many who have reached the same conclusion, though by diverse routes, and who are glad of it.

No one, I think, will dispute my first proposition: that, when there is physical disorder there is also some psychical disorder, and that, when there is psychical disorder, there is also some physical disorder. This is the true meaning of the phrase: *mens sana in corpore sano*, and of its complement: *mens insana in corpore insano*. Realisation of this is one of the elementary experiences of mankind: so elementary indeed, that it is overlooked by doctors who fail to see the physical signs in insanity, and the psychical disorder in what we call bodily disease. It is true that in some cases the physical aspect apparently predominates, as when we speak of "organic" disease; in others, the psychical as obviously predominates, and we say the patient is "mental." But there is a vast range of cases in which the psychical and physical disorders seem as it were nearly balanced. We dismiss such cases from our notice, calling them "functional." But that does not help the patient. It is to these cases, chiefly, that I would now direct attention, especially as for them the whole problem is easily resolved, if, without neglecting the physical, *we attach primary importance to the psychical aspect of the illness.*

Amongst the patients labelled cases of organic disease, we find the irascible man with aortic disease, the anxious man with a fatty myocardium, the hopeful youth with phthisis, and the hypochondriac with abdominal disease. At the other end of the scale, amongst the "mentals," we see the sweating, incontinent and mydriatic maniac with a full bounding pulse, and the desiccated, constipated, and myotic melancholic, with a slow, small, pulse. But, in the central group, we find those "functionals" who are the despair of the doctor and the joy of the charlatan—those who are cured by New Thought, Christian Science or Evangelical Conversion :—the migrainous with astigmatism : the vertiginous with middle ear catarrh : the asthmatic with no pulmonary or cardiac lesion : the hysterical dyspareunic with a misplaced uterus : the irritable and unstable old-young man with a big prostate: and the harassed doctor with flatulent dyspepsia or hyperchlorhydria. These are they in whom physical and psychical disorder are so nicely combined that diagnosis in ordinary terms is a matter of grave difficulty. But these are they in whom the inner man has the last word; if only it be spoken in time. If the golden moment pass by: if the patient be confirmed in his functional sins: such organic disease may develop as only the Surgeon amongst us (if even he) can remove. But, even then, even if what we call the "lesion" is triumphantly removed and put on a plate, the psychical disorder remains, and craves for what is seldom refused; yet more surgery, and more.

The *complete* picture of parallel physical and psychical disintegration is best seen in general paralysis of the insane; and we may say that here we have an instance of concomitant psychical and physical disorder produced without ever the option being offered to the Psyche. But I am not so sure.

I do not undervalue the importance of the spironema, but I have never seen a case of general paralysis—and I have seen a good many—in which slackening and degradation of moral and psychical control had not preceded the appearance of physical signs, if indeed, such psychical imbalance had not already preceded the acquisition of specific infection. So, even in the case of general paralysis, it is not unfair to say that the inner man has the last word before the die is cast that establishes progressive somatic and spiritual decay. The point that I am anxious to make, for it is fundamental, is this: that, because we meet with cases in which functional disorder of one kind or another has been followed by organic changes, irremovable by mental effort, we need not assume that there was *never* a stage in which organic change might have been averted, had only right functional adjustment been first established. Cowper put the situation admirably, so far as the physical and physical aspect of mental disease is concerned, when he wrote :—

> Faults in the life breed errors in the
> brain ;
> And these, reciprocally, those again.

Such, I think, is the play and interplay between what are called psyche and soma.

We need not, perhaps, pursue this train of thought farther, but if we enquire how organic changes can possibly be brought about in consequence of conscious or unconscious psychical states, we may find a link between brain and cord on the one hand, and between viscera and tissues on the other, not so much by way of " trophic" centres, or centres representing visceral activities, as by way of the sympathetic and parasympathetic systems, their cerebral and spinal connections and their control—in correspondence with emotional and other states—of those vasomotor, secretory and muscular mechanisms that do undoubtedly lie behind disease processes, whatever be the part played by micro-organisms or toxins in their production. One day, perhaps, the solar plexus will be allotted its rightful place in respect of psycho-physical precedence, and adjustment to the outer world.

What we must appreciate is that every case, whether in general or special practice, has a subjective pyschological interest and presents what may be called an objective psychological complex. It is true that we have no direct acquaintance with the minds of others: we appreciate their minds by the medium of signs: but equally we have no direct acquaintance with any form of disease in others: the disease is what we postulate to exist in the background of the signs.

We now come to a point that, I confess, is one not too willingly conceded by some of our most eminent teachers, although it is at once grasped by those who are more accustomed to think than to teach. In Medicine, those who teach, do not, as a rule, think. They repeat what they have been taught. Though the practice of our Art is to some extent empirical—based on experience, and afterwards explained by some theory that gives us the illusion of being rational—it is, nevertheless, very largely guided by the views we hold concerning the *nature* of disease, and the relation that we impute between what we call *mind* and *matter*. In other words, our notions concerning disease and its treatment are derived from our attitude towards certain metaphysical and philosophical problems. Time was when doctors of physic definitely studied philosophy in the broadest sense, and then systems of medicine were logically justified by current metaphysics. Nowadays we do not systematically study the foundations of knowledge and belief, and we ignore logic; but, nevertheless, medical doctrine is always, though unsystemically, expressed in terms of some form of metaphysical attitude, and usually in terms of some form that has been long discarded as inadequate by those whose business it is to occupy themselves with philosophy. Thus it is that many of our so-called advances in medicine are not so much the result of advances in actual discovery as expressions of a change of attitude towards the fundamental problems of life : a change of attitude that follows in the wake of metaphysical and philosophic thought. Considerations of this sort may not seem very relevant to questions of technique : as to, for example, whether a leg should be amputated by a circular or a flap method, and so forth. But they do become of extreme importance when we have to decide whether or no a patient with 'colitis' should be treated by laparotomy or by psychological methods. The man who holds one set of views will plump for appendicostomy, and will refuse to admit that psychological treatment can be useful : the man who holds to another will desire to postpone treatment by surgery until psychological treatment has been attempted. The one will say that, *because* the disease is organic, only surgery can help: the other will say that he will not be convinced the disease requires surgical aid until psychological investigation has proved useless. Each will define the terms used in his own way: the surgeon, by "organic," means something he thinks he should treat. The psychologist, by "psychical," means something he thinks he should treat. And so on. The man who does not believe in the supremacy of mind over matter will "go for" material remedies: the man who believes in that supremacy will avoid exclusive reliance on drugs and surgery until psychical resources have failed.

In further illustration of my point, let me remind you that, in the Far East, disease is generally regarded as the result of the abstraction of something spiritual from the body. Western races, on the whole, consider disease to be the expression of something added. In bygone centuries, this something added was, very frequently, a demon. To-day, this 'something added' is often something no less elusive and fictitious :—a toxin that no chemist can identify : a filter-passer that no microscopist can see. But, when a patient is constipated, a dose of castor oil or calomel is as efficacious, whether we give it with the intention to expel a demon or to eliminate a poison. Now, although we no longer believe in demons, official views in England concerning disease are still of a peculiar order : they are partly materialistic, and partly derived from the discarded metaphysics of scholastic realists. 'A' disease is officially something real, something to be studied as an objective entity : different diseases are said to be different kinds of natural objects, that can be studied in the same way as lions and tigers, postage stamps and coins, Conservatives and Socialists. This sort of talk, once current in Science, when Laws were supposed to govern the universe, and Forces like gravity to keep the heavenly bodies in place, is now obsolete, save only in medicine; and for those who are interested in modern psychology has little value. This is why, in the medical schools, where Victorian Science is still firmly embedded in medieval metaphysics, there is no clear teaching in respect of the psychological interest. One cannot accept the results of modern psycho-therapeutics so long as one believes that the only disease worth bothering about is something that "attacks" the patient, that makes a noise like a murmur, and that can be seen on a plate after death—when we have failed to cure the patient! People who think thus consider psychiatry a special method, that has nothing to do with really respectable medicine, but which may be employed, like violet rays, or a change of air, for those wretched cases "which have nothing the matter with them."

Now, roughly speaking, there are three sets of views which may be said to be held in medicine concerning the relation between body and mind. And each of these sets of psychological, philosophical, or metaphysical views corresponds to a definite set of views in respect of health and disease, and moulds, in respect of treatment, the whole attitude of those holding it.

We have, in the first place, the views of those who may be called materialists. Materialists—I am only speaking in the simplest terms—seek to explain the world as composed of one kind of stuff only: that which they call *matter* and which *moves*. The phenomena of mind are, for these people, produced by physical and chemical changes in the nervous system: consciousness is a product or function of protoplasm and nothing more. Doctors who think thus come to believe that, in disease, what is really important is the disturbance in fine or gross structure of the tissues or organs; while holding that disturbance of function is *always* a result of organic change, rather absurdly, they *call* "functional" those cases in which no structural change is detectable, and in which there is said to be no "organic disease." So they find these cases negligible, as annoying to their self-confidence!

If a person is disturbed in his mind without apparent adequate cause, it is either because he has organic or chemical change somewhere about him, or because he is a "functional case" not worth bothering about! If such people get well after treatment by surgery or drugs, it is proof that the materialistic view is correct! If they don't, they are hustled on one side as pestilent knaves, or consigned to a lunatic asylum! Anyway, they are got rid of, somehow or another, if indeed they do not commit suicide first. In the meantime, under influence of such notions as these, countless operations are performed, and countless treatments are carried through, on patients who *could* be successfully treated by what we will call psycho-therapy. Sometimes the result of the surgical treatment appears successful; but the method adopted is that of burning down the house to cook the pork chops, or of removing the tongue to cure the use of bad grammar!

A constipated lady, awaiting her husband's return from abroad, fears the detection of an amatory intrigue. She is uneasy: she has belly pain: she transfers her anxiety from her intrigue to her appendix, because her sister-in-law has just had appendicitis. A surgeon is called, and the appendix is removed, in an atmosphere of antiseptics and mutual admiration. It is found "congested." Reciprocal congratulations: six weeks in a nursing home: the lady and her lover forget each other: or the husband amuses himself elsewhere. All is well until the next amatory crisis, when the same surgeon is called in to remove adhesions, to take out the gall-bladder, or to fix the colon tautly. And so on. Nothing could be more satisfactory to all parties concerned.

Our second class of medical metaphysicians believe, confessedly or otherwise, that all we call material in this world is but an aspect, or consequence, of mental perspective, and that mind, or spirit, is the ultimate or only reality. Those who apply such views to the subject of healing, or who derive their practice from such views, comprise not only the spiritualists (true and false) but the Christian Scientists, and many psycho-analytical practitioners. They have much in common with the Neo-Platonists, and, to use an ambiguous form of expression, declare that, if all is well with the mind, soul, or spirit, all will be well with the body. It is idle to deny that many, who think thus and rule their lives accordingly, do adjust their reactions and escape many of those troublesome " functional " disorders that vex materialists who seek to allay, by treatment with blue lights or pink pills, the neurosis that follows on an uneasy conscience. It is idle to deny that the spiritual experiences of one kind or another, called conversion and so on, do rid life-long invalids, hypochondriacs, and neurotics of troubles for which they have suffered much at the hands of many physicians. But, on the other hand, we must admit that, when confronted with cases of cancer or of tuberculosis in an advanced stage, for example, the spiritualistic practitioners have either to wash their hands like Pilate—or to declare that the faith exhibited is insufficient for obtaining the result desired. At the same time, however, I am inclined to believe that what even a pathologist would call a case of organic disease may sometimes be cured by what we call psychological change. It is not good enough—to use a vulgarism—to say that, *because* a case is cured after a visit to Lourdes, it was never a case of organic disease ! To speak thus is to beg the whole question. Let me put it this way. When an unexpectedly good result is obtained after the administration of a simple drug in a confirmed and seemingly hopeless case, many surgeons and physicians will say : " Oh, yes ! But was it not the effect of suggestion ? "

The point is that the case recovered. To say " Suggestion " *explains* nothing. We might, with greater justification, say " Suggestion " when a laparotomy is performed successfully on a hysterical patient. When employing physical means we can never exclude a psychical effect, and, conversely, we can never exclude a " physical effect " when employing " psychical " means. If we give an enema, we are working on a low physical level; but we admit a psychical effect, as possible. If I say Abracadabra three times over, most people would say that I am only employing psychical means, and can therefore only hope for a psychical effect. Yet I am physically stimulating the auditory tract and its connections, just as definitely as does my friend who gives an enema so stimulate the rectum and its sympathetic and spinal connections. Merit, as between the materialists and the spiritualists, then, so far as pragmatic values are concerned, seems to be almost six of one and half-a-dozen of the other. This is perhaps why, in medicine, the *third* metaphysical school is so popular. This is the school of the dualists who find two substances, mind and matter, existing side by side. There are many kinds of dualisms, but the most popular doctrine amongst doctors is that of pyscho-physical parallelism, derived ultimately from the two-clock notion of Liebniz. Psycho-physical parallelism, as applied to the physiology and psychology of human beings, means that each physiological process has a concomitant psychological act or process as counterpart, and *vice versa.* It may be restricted, as many seem to restrict it, to the operations of the higher parts of the brain, or it may be applied to the whole of the nervous system—in which case we postulate that unconscious psychical processes accompany all physical nervous states of the spinal cord or nerves. Of course, too, this doctrine may be extended to cover all living things, and further, all material objects of perception whatsoever. Then we become what are called animists. But the restricted form of psycho-physical parallelism, which supposes mind and brain to work in "harmony", has a rather subtle practical value. Postulating that neither the one nor the other process has the upper hand, and that we cannot explain the connection between the two, it allows us to say that it is sometimes more convenient to tackle what we call the physical series—to rub in mercury in order that a gumma absorb: and sometimes better to tackle what we call the psychical—to employ suggestion or psycho-analysis in "appropriate" cases. This kind of facing-both-ways leads to what used to be called eclecticism: one kind of case is treated by drugs or surgery: another is sent to the asylum or the analyst. But, amongst eclectics, the functional neuroses tend to fall between two stools. This is the grave fault in the neurology of Hughlings Jackson and his pupils.

A quite different point of view—which I will call naturalistic—is, however, now coming into vogue. Those who adopt this outlook are neither 'materialistic' nor 'spiritualistic' in their interpretation of the world. They regard mind and matter as different names given to different aspects of what is but one. According to them we speak of matter when we see what is outside ourselves, and of mind when we refer to what we are subjectively. I am not at all sure that there is not a catch in this notion when we come to apply it to psychology and to physiology; but it is very useful in medicine. Conceive a man who is shut up in his study in the upper story of his house. He is in the world of pure mind. He becomes aware of discord, commotion, and discomfort. He looks out of the window, and he sees what is going on outside, in the world of matter. No explanation there. He leans out and sees the walls of his house, as does a man who regards his own body. All seems in order. He retires again and shuts the windows, but the disturbance and commotion, for which he sees no cause when he looks out of the window, continue. There is, as a matter of fact, internal discord in the kitchen—the region of the viscera—disturbing his emotional and better half, or sympathetic system —his wife, seated in her boudoir—the realm of the unconscious mind. We, called in as builders and surveyors, may try to restore order by getting the drains to go and the flues to draw, but we should do even better if, while doing all necessary plumbing work, as spiritual advisers we explained to our philosopher in his study that, did he exercise better control over his household, and pay proper attention to his marital duties, he would be able to pursue his studies to greater advantage. And such is the true *rôle* of the physician in cases of functional neurosis.

At any rate, this analogy is of some practical utility, and it does accord the last word, the casting vote, to the Inner Man—to what we call the 'Psyche.' For, had our philosopher better organised his household to begin with, the discord in the basement and the irritability of his wife would not have arisen, and the drains and chimneys would have been maintained in better working order.

There is, however, just one other trend of thought that is not at all unhelpful, and that would, I think, receive greater attention had it not such a definitely theological connotation. I mean the dualism of St. Thomas Aquinas, now the official system of the Roman Catholic Church, according to which primary matter is informed by spirit, of varying grade, so that each object, or substance, is composed of welded matter and spirit, and therefore is what it is. In this way the ultimate supremacy of spirit or mind is secured, while the dual aspect is not lost sight of. The non-theological view which comes nearest to this is the naturalistic one, just referred to. But clearly, on any shewing, for each of us, it is through our own mind that we come nearest to reality ; it is by own own mind that we must control our body ; and it is only by discussion of the various notions put forward that we can understand the issues, even if we may not be inclined to adopt any one solution.

If we now turn to what are called practical considerations in respect of the management—not of what we call organic cases, and not of what we call "mental" cases—we will find that in practice a method found useful in respect of asthmatic, of migrainous, and of vertiginous and neuralgic persons, of "functional" cardiac and dyspeptic patients, of mucous colitis cases, of the sexual sufferers, the prostatic cases, and the anxiety, compulsion, and hysterical neurotics, will be found increasingly useful in respect of what we usually consider as purely "mental" or purely "organic" cases. Nay: it will be found useful even in the management of a patient with a broken leg, at any rate so far as his insomnia and his contentment are concerned. And, does not that stand for much? I have known an ununited fracture of the tibia to heal, after months of suffering, only when a conjugal difficulty was dissipated in the courts.

This is the method. We must, in the first place, institute a complete physical examination, appraising the disorder of function manifestly present, and then estimating, so far as is possible, the organic change in the organs that are not functioning well. This is, or should be, the normal clinical procedure. But something more is wanted. We must form some idea of the original efficiency of the organ or structure in respect of which complaint is made. We then find, for example, that the migrainous and the neuralgic persons have usually some facial asymmetry, or some morphological defect: the asthmatics have imperfectly developed nares, epiglottides and larynges, and, if we dissect them, not only poor chests, but lungs that are imperfectly developed *qua* lobes. Our tinnitus and vertigo patients have poor external ears: our dyspeptics, dilated or ptotic stomachs: our cardiac cases small and pendent, or large and pushed-up hearts: our hypochondriacs and our colitis cases have long mesenteries, mobile colons, mobile kidneys, and the like. Our sexual neurotics have small, or misplaced uteri; varicoceles, phimoses, pendent scrotums and so on. Our spinal neurasthenics, as well as many others, have rudimentary spinae bifidae, and a tendency to pes cavus and hammer toe—because the terminal spine is imperfectly developed. Nay: even our rheumatoid and arthritic patients, often enough, have digits and limbs with which there is something wrong from the point of view of the sculptor, just as do many insane patients exhibit the most extraordinary skin peculiarities—strong evidence that the part of the epiblast from which the neural tissues are formed is not what it should be. All this comprises the study of *organ inferiorities*, as it is called—our philosopher has chosen a jerry-built house—and the organ inferiorities we notice in the neurotic are either in connection with the organs working badly—as when we see the small penis and long prepuce of the boy who wets his bed—or afford inferential evidence of other organ defect—as when the external auricle is malformed in a tinnitus patient—or suggest a widespread deficiency, as do the segmentally distributed skin defects found in association with neurasthenia.

In the same way, many of the women with a "neurotic abdomen" have a fissured tongue, so that we can postulate a Meckel's diverticulum or something of that sort, while a neurasthenic miner with lumbago probably has a sacralized fifth lumbar vertebra that has been jarred.

The importance of such observations lies in this, that they reveal either constitutional or local inferiority to which may be transferred an emotional feeling that rightly pertains to something in the psychical life. To give a simple illustration. The actress with astigmatism, who desires not to appear on a certain occasion (because she fears her psychical nose will be out of joint) develops a headache (due to eye strain, she says) that gives her an *excuse* while satisfying her unacknowledged and unacknowledgeable desire to vindicate her own importance. We may give her glasses: but her headaches will continue, on suitable occasions! Our war experiences help us to understand this. The shell-shocked man with 'cold feet,' who durst not acknowledge his cowardice, became deaf if he had a perforated drum: blind, if he had astigmatism or squint: paralysed in his legs, if he had spinal inferiority with hammer toes; and wetted the bed if he had a varicocele and a long foreskin. So it is only the woman who dislikes her husband who, with a retroflexed uterus, or a prolapsed ovary, suffers dyspareunia. She has no dyspareunia with her lover. Where there is a will not to do, there is always a way of escape from doing what should be done, and what we *know* ought to be done.

But this is going too fast. Having completed the physical examination, in the way I suggest, we must proceed to examination of the pyschical situation. There are various methods of performing this, but none can be properly utilised unless what is called the New Psychology be understood, at any rate in outline. The old psychology was a study of mind, based largely upon introspection, and so derived from investigation of intelligent, normal, and cultivated persons. It was governed largely by the assumption that the mind, like the brain and spinal cord, responds to stimulus in a predetermined sort of way. We tap the patella tendon, and the knee jerks. We present a stimulus to the mind, and we observe a normal response. So the psychical response was formerly held to be determined by the stimulus. *Mais nous avons changé tout cela.* The new psychology, largely based upon study of the neurotic, implies another theory.

We examine the response—that is to say, the behaviour—of the patient, and then work back, seeking, not for the sort of stimulus that would or should make what we think a 'normal' so act, but for the tendency that the patient is seeking to gratify by his, to us, odd behaviour. Thus, a busy man complains of strange cardiac sensations, or tells us he is irritable at home, especially with his wife. We, simple souls, would once have told him that he was overworked, and advised him to take his wife for a week-end to Brighton. Nowadays we find he is afraid of not carrying through successfully some business enterprise, and so seeks an excuse, in the state of his heart, for abandoning it ! Moreover, he has just spent a week-end at Brighton with his best typist, and is trying to justify his infidelity by finding such fault with his wife as will reconcile his conscience to the commission of acts of which he is ashamed ! Probably, too, he left his fountain pen behind him at Brighton, and thinks his memory is failing !

Three psychological categories have to be taken into account if we would understand fully the " neurotic " or " functional " patient. There is, in the first place, the acknowledged, or unacknowledged, unsettled conflict or perplexity in the patient's mind.

Secondly, there is to be recognised a guiding tendency that is the result of past experience, ancestral as well as individual, for which satisfaction is somehow sought, in respect of every situation that arises. Thirdly, there is the past life history, determining *why* the tendency—the life-line—is as it is, and why the satisfaction is not *directly* sought ; the *reason* why it is sought alternatively, or, so to speak, vicariously. And, on the physical side, there is the relevant organ-inferiority that offers the excuse for organisation of a " functional illness," and is so eagerly seized upon as the peg whereon is hung the vestment we wish to discard, so that we have not the burden of wearing it ; or that we wish to wear, and dare not : or that looks to us like a spectre in the dark.

There are almost as many methods of elucidating these matters clinically as there are theories of the mechanisms concerned. The chief theories and methods are those of Freud : of Jung : and of Adler.

Freud and his pupils, in method, rely largely upon the study of dreams, and of errors in speech, in memory, and in conduct ; and they seek above all to revive the earliest and most buried memories of childish life. Jung has devoted time and labour to the revival of hidden memories by the use of what is called word-association, as well as by free association and talk ; Adler comes quickly to the point, states at once to the patient the outline of the problem, and then pursues developments.

The reason for these variations in technique is given in the respective theoretical views of the three great men I have referred to.

Freud finds the primary conflict in the sexual sphere, and deems the nature of the patient's reactions to all problems to be determined by his early sexual experiences, and especially by his attitude towards, and his experiences with his Father and Mother. Sex-life in the past, is the Freudian explanation in a phrase. Jung finds the problem to be that of satisfactions of the *libido* here and now; and by *libido* means something far more than sexual desire. "Satisfaction in the present" may be said to be the formula of Jung. Adler finds ambition, the desire to assert superiority, to gain one's own ends, the great motive which, once baulked, leads to neurosis. Goal attainment is the Adlerian *cliché*.

There is truth in each of these points of view, without doubt. We may say that each is, on occasion, most convenient. None is to be regarded as final. When the complaint made to the doctor (whether it be of colitis, of vertigo, or of migraine, for example) lies chiefly within the physical sphere, and is obviously a complaint of deranged physical function, then, without doubt, the factor of organ-inferiority, stressed by Adler, is of much importance as is the play of the superiority motive in the psychical sphere. When the *complaint* is psychical, and there is an obvious sexual nexus, great help is derived from investigation of the

Father-Mother relationships of early life, as stressed by Freud. When the trouble arises from what is very, very far from uncommon, a conflict in the sphere of the religious and intellectual emotions, then the teachings of Jung are particularly valuable. In no case can any element be overlooked; in some, all three points of view have a measure of validity, so curiously interwoven and so complex is the psychical state of the neurotic. It follows, almost as a matter of course, that each physician tends to develop a technique in terms of his own life history, in investigation no less than in treatment. But, for the general practitioner, and in relation to the class of case we are chiefly discussing, I think it is the technique, and in great measure the theory, of Adler—the theory that all conflicts reduce to a conflict between the superiority claim and the inferiority realization—that is the most useful, at the outset.

Equally it is clear that investigation demands, on the part of the physician, something much more than acquaintance with the mere facts of medicine as taught in the schools. Unless there is a pretty wide knowledge of pyschical types, of life-situations, of trends of thought, and of human nature in all its aspects, psychological investigation is impossible. The wider our own personal experiences, the greater our own knowledge of the human heart and mind as dissected in art and literature, and the fuller our acquaintance with the views held in respect of religious and philosophical problems, as well as of ethical difficulties, the more successful will our efforts be. Perhaps that is the meaning of the maxim that, at fifty, one is either a fool or a physician! The important point is that for each neurotic there is, not only some immediate problem which is not being decided, and in respect of which there is a conflict, an attempted compromise or some abortive repression into the limbo of the unconscious, some putting away of what is unpleasant or unwelcome—there is also a special attitude towards life in general which is adopted in face of almost every problem of adjustment, whether in connection with the family, the school, the opposite sex, society, one's profession, and religious, or irreligious inclinations. This attitude, however coloured, is generally one of indecision in practice, of irresolution, of procrastination and evasion, so that the conflict is never settled, and compensations for what is denied, satisfactions which are not openly claimed, excuses for what shames, insurances for what is feared—in fact, a whole cloud of "mechanisms" and arrangements—are set up. So the child complains of stomach-ache when, for some reason of which he guards the secret, he does not want to go to school! Such is a simple case, and in practice, none is quite so simple as this. Yet there are certain very common correlations, as we shall see.

Now, while the first object of the psychical inquisition is to lay bare all such mechanisms and arrangements, just as, in the clinical wards, we seek to picture the organic arrangements, the metabolic disturbances, and the microbic infections that lie behind the manifest symptoms of which the patient complains, the *second* object is that, after the picture has been made clear to the doctor, the patient himself may come to understand his or her own psychical mechanisms and the reason for his or her physical behaviour in this or that fashion or on this or that occasion. Then the therapeutic end comes to be fulfilled. To use a phrase that has perhaps been abused, the patient assumes conscious control of the disturbing unconscious factors, and, if the conflict is rightly resolved, well-being returns, all being done that rightly can be done, to assist, by physical means, the resumption of control, by the nervous system, of those visceral functions whereof disorder has been the motive for advice being sought.

The Neo-Platonic scheme of Plotinus is very usefully borne in mind at this stage. Let us picture the self as of three levels. The highest, or Nous, corresponding to our highest and most conscious intelligence, presides over a lower level, that of the soul (in the old terminology) and *that* over the soma, or body. Suppose we parallel this, and speak of the conscious mind and brain. on the highest level; the unconscious mind and sympathetic system, on the next; and the viscera and animal life on the lowest. We then have a not unhelpful conception. Not very much unlike our analogy of the philosopher in his study! Each level depends upon control from the higher level, and may be disturbed by disorder in the one below it. And, I need not emphasize how, according to Plotinus, the highest balance and harmony is attained only so far as the Nous, or highest level, is in accord with the highest perfection and intelligence of all. This, it may be said, is only, in other words, the doctrine of the Christian Scientist and the Salvation Army Evangelist. Perhaps, but it is also, in effect, the doctrine, though differently expressed, of Plato, of Confucius, and of Buddha.

Now, before again touching on what are usually called really practical details I would like to suggest as true, what all can easily verify, that certain forms of psychical distress are more or less definitely correlated with certain physical complaints. The man or woman who complains of migraine or of trigeminal neuralgia is, I think, without exception, placed in some situation that gives rise to an unexpressed, or unrecognised emotion of, to use Adler's words, rage and humiliation. The vertiginous neurotic is one who has constantly with him the fear of falling: morally, socially, or financially. Patients with tinnitus are generally patients who refuse to listen to some imperative call and the kind of noise of which they complain often gives a key to the difficulty. Those who are neurotic asthmatics are obsessed by an urge towards economy (not always in respect of money), and who regret expenditure. The miser in a novel always wheezes! Whilst patients with true or false angina are angry and resentful "at heart" the ordinary case of cardiac neurosis suffers from fear, from anxiety, and, very often, from unacknowledged or unsatisfied sexual desire.

It is odd how common phraseology helps us. We speak of a maddening head-ache, say we feel sick about something, have anger in our heart, or are in a piddling funk. These verbal combinations indicate those psychical correlatives of physical states which were perfectly well known to the Hebrew prophets and psalmists.

Nay: there is far more truth than we acknowledge in the Graeco-Roman correlation between the bile, black bile, lymph and blood, and the emotions symbolized when we speak of being liverish, splenetic, phlegmatic, and sanguine.

The flatulent dyspeptic has usually reason to resent, or even loathe, that which he is compelled, or thinks himself compelled to swallow: constipation is associated with sexual repression and avarice: diarrhoea, sometimes with a desire to be rid of this or that; and so-called colitis, not so much with a repression of sexuality as with an unsatisfied desire for sexual gratification. The physiological explanation of this is that the colon (though not the small intestine) is associated, *via* the sacral autonomic system, with the sexual viscera. Similar sympathetic associations can be traced in some other cases, but this is obvious, and the transference of nervous tension can be easily understood. Sexual *neuroses* are commonly associated, I think, with remorse or self-dissatisfaction in connection with sexual action. The man who is impotent with a prostitute may be so protecting himself against sin and infection; the syphilophobic has always, I think, fear or remorse for past or present wrong doing in his mind, and is trying indirectly to satisfy his conscience, or protect himself in respect of what he has not the moral courage to renounce. Paralysis of the functional type carries often the same kind of explanation, and the psychical element in sciatica, that *is* sciatica, is often very clear. It is generally the expression of a desire to shirk a duty or avoid a danger, and is associated with a sacro-lumbar organ-inferiority that can be demonstrated by X-rays. Of course, once more, I am only drawing the broadest outlines, but I will narrate one case in partial detail. A middle-aged man consulted a surgeon for pain in the back. The surgeon found a lipoma in the region indicated, but refrained from removing it when he heard that the pain only occurred on certain occasions (such as entering a crowded drawing-room) and was associated with faintness. The patient was brought to me. It was soon clear that this man, on four or five occasions during his life, had endured what he thought unmerited hard luck, financially and in marital affairs. On each occasion he tried, unwisely and from real cowardice, to put a brave face before the world, and hide his griefs. At the time of his visit to me he had made a fortune, and had married, as he thought, happily at last. But his wife had suddenly become a hopeless invalid. He denied any early associations that might have explained his history, and we went on talking. Suddenly he flushed and sweated, and said, "Doctor, you are right. When at school I was thrashed for a lie I never told : I thought of suicide and fainted in chapel the next day. It is *that* pain, *that* faintness, that I have ever since suffered when I have felt punished unfairly."

After this conversation, the pain never returned. Moreover, the lipoma disappeared. Was the lipoma a result of concentration, unconsciously, on the painful memory ? Or, was the lipoma an excuse for its unconscious persistence ?

But now, the physical and psychical diagnosis being made, if not in detail, at any rate in such broad outline as is possible at an early stage, let us turn specifically to the therapeutic management of the case. Let the patient understand that there is both a physical and a psychical side to his unwellness, and let us outline the physical treatment necessary. It may of course be (and in eye, ear, and other special cases often is) necessary to enlist the aid of a specialist friend. Such a friend, unless he is sympathetically inclined towards psychological investigation, is only too certain to put a damaging spoke in the wheel, effectually, and at an early stage. Even if he be sympathetically inclined, he may, by exceeding the limits of his own province, do more harm than good. Under such circumstances I would advise you to be careful to ask for just what you do want: namely, an opinion on the physical condition and too, one given without any discussion of the nervous element and its importance. During the last year or two I have been unusually fortunate in having been able to rely upon the co-operation of my friend, Mr. Norman Fleming, in matters ophthalmological, and we have been able to secure some extremely happy results, in migrainous and other cases, each giving due regard to the importance of the other's share in the task of integrating health. Whether the full psychological treatment itself be undertaken by the general practitioner, or by a physician who has paid special attention to the subject, is another matter. So far as is possible, the physician chosen (if one be chosen) should be one who has general knowledge and sympathies (as has Adler), rather than a specialist psycho-analyst: at any rate for the class of patient we have now chiefly in mind. It is essential that he be competent in the diagnosis and treatment of 'physical' maladies. But I am all in favour of the general practitioner retaining full treatment in his own hands, if he feels himself competent and confident, and has had experience. A physician consulted, as "second opinion", may advise helpfully *once*, but cannot as a rule do much more, unless the psychical treatment is confided to him as wholeheartedly as is the conduct of an operation to a surgeon. It may be, and often is, advisable that this course be followed. If so, let it be followed without reserve. It is impossible for intimate conversations to be held with the physician and the practitioner alternately: it is generally impossible for confidences to be repeated, and, above all, if full conduct is given to the physician, there is the less danger of the wearying and frustrating intervention of relatives who, too often, are predisposing and exciting morbific agents! In a word, if the patient's confidence is to be gained, it must be deserved, and kept. There are some other points to be considered. Even a superficial analysis is exhausting to the physician, and therefore interviews should be frequent, and so far as is possible, consecutive, though sometimes much may be done in less time than is usually required.

The psychological examination and treatment of the young is a special matter, to which not enough attention is usually given. The advice of a physician of experience is here usually required, since any action necessary is not so much directed to the patient as to the modification of the circumstances of his life in a way that is not usually palatable to a misguided and obstinate parent.

On the other hand, prolonged attempts at psychical investigation are seldom very useful when the patient is over fifty or fifty-five, though something can be achieved sometimes, if tried in the right way. But, what I may call psychotherapy has its fullest scope between the ages of perhaps twenty and forty.

The aim of the physician must be, then, to help the patient to know himself, and to understand the mechanism and arrangements that he has unconsciously constructed around his disturbed area of conflict. He must be led to see where is the difficulty : that compromise and indecision are no solution. He must be shewn, or rather led, to see that adjustment to the family, and to society, and to ultimate problems must be made. But the solution must not be dictated. The patient must herein minister to himself; he must work out his own salvation. And again I would say that the method of Adler, which involves early categorical diagnosis on the part of the physician, and early statement to the patient, is the best: at any rate if the patient is one inclined to cry: "What must I do to be saved?" If, that is, he is really desirous of freeing himself from what as yet he has only partly confessed to himself.

The method of Freud presents special difficulties in the cases of which we have been speaking; it requires many interviews, and there is, first the technical difficulty of what is called resistance, and secondly, that of transference. Resistance is met with when communication cannot be opened up freely, and when interviews are postponed and avoided. The very nature of Freudian analysis often provokes this in England, at any rate, for the relation of the inquiry to the urgent complaints is far from obvious to a patient who comes complaining of what appears to him to be a bodily illness. With Adler's method, the relation of the physical symptoms to a psychical state can be confidently pointed out at once. Again, transference, by which is meant the development of an attractive or repellent emotional state in regard to the physician, is better avoided, as under Freudian analysis it is not. Under Adler's technique, with less insistence on the sexual factor in any case, and with hardly any in some, the feeling that the patient comes to entertain towards the physician is, as it should be, free from embarrassment to either. But it may still be desirable that the physician be one who, if not an actual stranger, is at any rate not a participant in the social life enjoyed by the patient. His attitude should be, if if not that of a pedagogue or a priest, at any rate one that involves a certain degree of apartness, of authority, and of prestige.

One word in conclusion. If a single formula is required in which to summarise the teachings of Freud, of Jung, and of Adler, it may, I think be found in the teaching of the famous sermons of Bishop Butler. Butler reduced the authorities in the polity of the soul to two: conscience and self-love. The term self-love covers equally the pleasure-principle of Freud, the libido of Jung, and the superiority-aim of Adler. By conscience we may understand the countervailing impulses, present to us all, that tend in certain circumstances to inhibit self-gratification. The recent theory of Blondel, involving discrimination between 'la conscience claire' and 'la conscience morbide' approximates of course closely to this; but for a Frenchman the word 'conscience' has not the ethical significance conveyed to an Englishman. I do not propose, however, to discuss or consider whether a theory of conscience (in the English rather than the French sense) should be based upon the doctrine of an implanted intuition, or whether by conscience we should understand the operation of the sum of early teachings and experiences. But *we* all know what conscience is: there is no man, woman or child who has not experienced it, and we have all seen expression of its workings even in a pet dog. So, after all, there is common ground alike for Freud and for those who explain all physical and psychical ill as consequences of the Fall. In great part of what the new psychologists have to say, we are only learning anew, and in a new language, what was known centuries ago, but what, in the pride of modern scientific research, we have too carelessly forgotten.

And, if we read again the story of how Nathan the prophet dealt with David, we will realise that there are methods quicker and more searching than even those of Adler himself. Not a dissection: not a vivisection: but an operation, the reduction of a dislocation, is what is required when psychotherapy is undertaken.

Two further points. The scope of the psychological interest in general practice is immense. Nothing could be more deplorable than diffusion of the idea that the psychological investigation of the neuroses means the discussion of sexual topics with young girls; and psycho-therapy, the recommendation of fornication. I recently heard a celebrated surgeon say: "Freud: oh! that's the feller who says copulation is the cure for everything!" No: when the sexual complexes are predominant, the patient suffers, not because he or she is not physically gratified, but because, for one reason or another, a wrong attitude has been taken up in respect of the practical and ethical problems involved in Human Life and by Human Conduct.

And this leads us towards the second point. Now-a-days we are far too apt to "explain" all tendencies and aberrations of emotion and conduct as determined by and dependent upon the nature and balances of our internal gland-secretions. It is true that, in clinical medicine, by administering certain substances such as thyroid gland or pituitary, we can sometimes effect wonderful changes in mental and physical functioning. But it is no less true, and of even greater importance that, by persistence in certain emotional reactions and by the deliberate continuance of certain forms of conduct, we can modify, first, the functional activities and, secondly, the actual organization of those glands which, by materialists, are supposed to dictate our emotional responses and our conscious endeavours. Frankenstein's Monster, in the end, slew his Master. But it was Frankenstein himself who first created the Monster, and on whom the ultimate responsibility for his own destruction rested. In everyday life, it is the Monsters of our own creation who slay not only ourselves but our children—unto the third and fourth generation—for the effective gland-balance in the child is, often enough, as it were but an expression of the positive or negative psychological and ethical trends of the parent as consciously exercised and developed.

II

MIGRAINE AND ITS ALLIES[1]

The subject of this lecture has been chosen, in the first place, because it is one of intrinsic importance. A vast amount of suffering is endured by the migrainous and, moreover, the migrainous entail much discomfort on those associated with them. But, in the second place, this topic has been chosen for discussion because it is one that is too often dealt with superficially and inadequately. It is true that of late years ophthalmic skill and the free use of coal-tar derivatives have afforded some relief to the sufferers, yet it is hardly too much to say that still, as thirty years ago, migraine is often looked upon as at once incurable and almost unworthy of notice by the physician.

[1] A Lecture delivered at the North-East London Post Graduate College. 1924.

A third reason is that, in discussing migraine and some allied conditions, opportunity occurs for availing ourselves of a method of approach that will, I am confident, come to be applied in the near future with ever-increasing success and profit.

When dealing with one who is ill, or who complains of being ill, the physician too often makes use of only one of three methods of inquiry that are available.

He may concern himself with the obvious disturbances of physical function that are present. This is the symptomatological method, of late too much neglected by orthodox authority, but recently revived by Sir James Mackenzie.

Or, believing that no disease is worthy of serious attention that has not what is called an organic basis, the physician may occupy himself almost exclusively with the investigation of the signs of change or defect in structure. This is the method of the organicist school; it is based upon the study of the physical signs found during life and the structural changes found after death.

Lastly, there is the line of attack of those who attach cardinal importance to disturbances of the psyche—to the neglect sometimes of all evidences of organic defect or change—and who, in psychical disorder, find the universal explanation of physiological dysharmonies.

This is the method of certain psychological schools and one that, in an extreme form, is adopted by Christian Scientists, and by those who think to conquer disease by imagining it not to be present. Now the fully-equipped physician must recognise the value in each case—though in each case in different measure—of each of these three methods. Confronted with disease, he must investigate, in each case, the present disorder of function—of physiological function, that is: the present defect or change in organs or in tissues—themselves the expression of disorder in internal or vegetative function: and the present psychological state, or mode of psychological reaction, to present external realities.

Only thus can the "present state" of a patient be fully appreciated.

But the physician must be prepared to do more: he must consider not only the psychological history of the individual but his physiological life-history—his past physiological reactions—and his organic life-history—as indicated by the morphology of his organs and tissues and the manifest anthropological and endocrine types: in a word, by his line of organic development as well as by his pathological state—physical and psychological.

Only thus can the physician comprehend in what manner, and as a result of what chains of circumstance, has the "present state"—physical, physiological, and psychological—come to be; or, how it is that *this* person is reacting as he *now* does to the circumstances in which he finds himself—circumstances in respect of which the physician will take care, of course, to be fully advised.

Now, if we apply ourselves after this fashion—at once analytical and synthetic—to the study of the migrainous, we find that, not only is there close correspondence between the details of the paroxysms in different persons, but that there is singular accord in the psychological states, in the modes of psychological reaction throughout life, in the physiological constitutions, and in the physical types that are brought before us. Notably do we meet with what Adler would call similar organ-inferiorities, and notably do we discover certain psychological failings, as well as, perhaps, certain psychological qualities that are not lightly to be depreciated.

What do we understand by migraine? We mean, I think, a peculiar and paroxysmal—and therefore recurrent—headache, that is usually, but not invariably, referred to one side of the head only. What may be called a typical paroxysm of migraine is best described as passing in three stages. In the first, there is a vague but generalised feeling of malaise, during which various subjective ocular phenomena are noticed. The so-called fortification zigzags are well-known: sometimes there is definite hemianopia: muscæ volitantes are commonly seen. With the onset of the second stage there are generalised vaso-motor disturbances, often enough: pallor, tremblings, and the like; and headache ensues. The headache is variously described: it becomes intense, incapacitating: the sufferer is forced to withdraw to a darkened room, to lie down, and to wait for its passing. In the third stage the headache reaches its maximum of intensity, and there may be violent vomiting or retching, generally bilious.

Suddenly, when after violent retching a moment of utter helplessness and prostration is experienced, the headache may pass completely away. Then the patient will sleep; and, after an hour or two, he may be himself again; perhaps even more cheerful than he has been for days.

Such is a typical and violent attack, as experienced during the life-period of sexual activity ; let us say, between sixteen and fifty. During the life-period that we may call pre-sexual —from early childhood to adolescence —the attacks are usually, by observers, recognised as bilious attacks—sometimes indeed, as fits of temper. In the third period of life—that of sexual wane—the attacks are less " organised " and vomiting is infrequent. In more than one respect the attacks then remind us of the Cheshire cat's grin, which remained when the cat itself had faded away.

To diagnose migraine should not be difficult ; that is to say, as to diagnose is commonly understood now-a-days. But the achievement of the nominal diagnosis is only a step in the direction of the complete and Hippocratic diagnosis. Two cautions are, however, necessary. Not a few migrainous children have been " explored " as the subjects of an " acute " or " chronic " abdomen ; many more have been carelessly treated as "bilious." And, when the climacteric has been passed, headaches that are very migrainous in character are sometimes associated with "true" uræmia, or, more commonly, with a retention of urea that seems to depend upon errors in diet and upon hepatic and renal inadequacy. Again, true migraine in early adult life often passes insensibly into the headache of hyperpiesia.

However, even in the middle or sexual period of life, all attacks are not as just described. Sometimes they may be said to abort; sometimes they succeed each other rapidly during days, or even weeks, so that we think of a migrainous *status* comparable to the *status epilepticus*: sometimes they are anomalous, commencing with trigeminal neuralgia; sometimes they blend with trigeminal neuralgia; and, sometimes they alternate with paroxysms of such neuralgia.

In very severe paroxysms, aphasia is not uncommon; temporary monoplegia, usually brachial, is sometimes experienced by young subjects, and a multiplicity of vaso-motor disorders has been described. One feature is important; during the attack the kidneys may act but very scantily, and with remission of the headache there may be a copious flow of colourless urine of low specific gravity.

Here again points of contact with the more or less permanent arterial spasm of hyperpiesia are established. I do not propose to discuss at any length orthodox theories of migraine. It is obvious enough that during the paroxysm there is widespread vaso-motor disorder; and there is not a little evidence that, in part at least, this is unilateral, or asymmetrical in distribution,

A recent writer, I think with reason. incriminates at once the solar plexus and the brain, but invokes, with less justification, that very present help in time of trouble, protein or anaphylactic shock, as the factor that disturbs the harmony that should obtain between these structures (*Schw. Med. Woch.*, May 19th, 1921).

Other writers have thought that turgescence of the pituitary gland may play a part in the physiological mechanism of migrainous attacks ; and it is possible that such is the case.

An important theory is that of Wollaston, who localised the " brain-storm " in the optic thalamus, a view adopted and expanded by Liveing, and which we can the better appreciate now that we recognise correlation between emotion-states and thalamic-states.

Still, all these explanations and notions carry us but a little way ; and to speak of fatigue, of worry, of anxiety, of excesses, of indiscretions in diet, of constipation and so forth, though necessary and important, is not sufficient, if we would really get to the bottom of the trouble and understand its origins.

Who are the people that are migrainous ? A remarkable fact—and it may be a solace to any one of our readers who is migrainous—is that quite a number of the sufferers is found among the intellectual and intelligent. Not a few distinguished medical men, and many celebrated physicists, astronomers, and philosophers have been migrainous, and have left us illuminating accounts of their sufferings. These people, though actively engaged in their respective pursuits, have been as a rule men regarded as thinkers rather than as "doers." They have been given to abstract thought, and to the pursuit of general ideas and, though not prone to emotional expression, have been credited, or discredited, with lack of feeling. In a word, never quite common place, or ordinary, in their own spheres of life the migrainous are people who, in Jung's phraseology, are to be regarded as *introverts*, and, moreover, usually as *thinking introverts*.

Perhaps men suffer more frequently from true migraine than do women, but not a few women are migrainous, and they too may be recognised as strongly introverted.

On the physical side, the resemblances are no less marked. Generally, the migrainous are of robust physique; they come of long-lived families; and live long. An endocrinologist would not, as a rule, say that any deficiency of the gonads exists—the migrainous are not sexually deficient—and would be inclined to postulate at least a pituitary sufficiency. The patients are energetic, and industrious; they possess, usually, greater rather than lesser cranial capacity, and are long-headed as a rule.

Physiologically, they are not of what old physicians would have called the lymphatic or phlegmatic temperament; the vaso-motor system is, with them, in unstable rather than in stable equilibrium, however self-contained and reserved may be their apparent attitude towards events.

On close examination, in both the migrainous and in those who suffer from paroxysmal trigeminal neuralgia, a certain organ-inferiority is generally obvious.

That is to say, there is a more or less definite facial asymmetry manifested by asymmetrical play of facial muscles, by deviation of the nasal septum, by lack of balance between ocular muscles and, sometimes, by dental irregularities and the like. Slight degrees of hypermetropia or of myopia, associated with astigmatism, or with imbalance, are nearly always present and, as a rule, the error of refraction is itself asymmetrical.

The importance of this "organ-inferiority" is very great. Let us remember how, during the War, those who under strain and stress became functionally blind, deaf, or dumb, were always found amongst those who, before the time of shock, had displayed either congenital or acquired "inferiority" in respect of the organs of sight, of hearing, or of speech, respectively.

The relation of this organ-inferiority to the actual paroxysm is threefold. The defect, as in the case of imbalance, may be an actual cause of cerebral exhaustion, by reason of the efforts made to overcome the resulting disability. Or, as in the case of an hypertrophied turbinate, organ-defect may be a factor in the production of symptoms and at the same time a result of long-continued functional irregularity; thus maintaining a vicious circle. Again, organ-defect may become the excuse, seized upon by the psyche, as we shall see, for the maintenance of a persistent psychological attitude. But, always is it of vital importance in treatment that the organ-inferiority be remedied or compensated, so far as in our power.

The ordinary treatment of migrainous persons—apart from the compensation or removal of organ inferiority—consists in the regulation of the daily life in accordance with the best principles of hygiene, and in the prescription of various medicines to be taken, during the attacks, for the relief of headache. Luminal if given regularly may succeed for a time in apparently staving off attacks. I do not propose to discuss these points in detail, but one item is very important. Any glasses prescribed by the ophthalmic surgeon for constant wear should be assumed immediately on waking in the morning. That the error of refraction, or the muscular imbalance, is trifling is no excuse for infringement of this rule : in dealing with migraine the very little counts often for very much.

But, however skilful the ophthalmic surgeon, and however meticulous the general treatment, although relief from the actual paroxysms may be obtained, the patient does not become *well*, unless the psychological situation is elucidated and adjusted. I say nothing of the merits of peptone-therapy and the like : in my opinion any effects produced by this and similar methods are magical and not fundamental. Attention of body and mind is diverted into new channels, perhaps : but as much may be procured in half a dozen different ways.

Something more than diversion of attention, physical or psychical, and something more than the comfortable words of Coué are required if real and lasting benefit is to be secured.

It is not a little odd that, so far as is known, neither Freud nor Jung has devoted attention to the psychology of the migrainous. Adler certainly has, in his recently published *Individual Psychology* (Kegan Paul, 1924) which should be read by all who are interested in the questions on which I propose to touch. But perhaps the most skilful treatment of the subject is that offered, albeit perhaps unintentionally, in *The Helpmate*: that fine novel written by Miss May Sinclair, herself a very competent philosopher and psychologist. Those who read this book, and who appreciate the circumstances under which the hero—if hero be the word—suffers from headache, will the more easily follow what Adler has written, not only concerning the migrainous, but in respect of those who suffer trigeminal neuralgia.

Now, if the present psychological state of any one who seeks relief from migraine be investigated, it will be found that, *although the patient himself will at first deny the fact,* yet always the mental content, in the neighbourhood of the paroxysms, or during their persistence, is one that, in Adler's phrase, is coloured by repressed "rage and humiliation."

The sufferer will protest that he feels no rage or humiliation, but, if pressed, or moved to speak freely, will admit annoying circumstances that would perhaps provoke feelings of "rage and humiliation" in anyone endowed with less control and of a coarser nature than himself!

Here is the key to the situation: the migrainous person asserts his or her "superiority"; hints that he or she is the victim of circumstances or of the foolishness or worse of others; takes no decisive steps to end or adjust a situation that is frankly intolerable —and suffers from migraine, either in face of, or in anticipation of, failure to gain his or her end: to impose his or her "superiority." Blame for failure is then transferred by the subject from where it is justly due, to the organ-inferiority, which is " the cause of the headache."

Let me give an hypothetical case that will serve as illustration. A professional man, who, with some justice feels that he is a square peg in a round hole, has to perform some task which is perhaps not congenial, and in respect of which he dreads failure, feeling perhaps the while that he could much better do something more difficult. Migraine ensues at the critical moment, and an excuse is ready to hand. Of course, he would not have failed had he not had one of his headaches! A well known *physician*, now dead, has given a wonderful account of his own sufferings and how once an attack came on when he had to *operate* for appendicitis.) Another is passed over for promotion in favour of a junior whom he deems inferior to himself —perhaps justly. Again, migraine or neuralgia: sick leave; and perhaps resignation. Worry may be admitted as a cause of the headache: but it is " worry " due to domestic affairs, his wife's health, or what not—anything but his own real or feared incapacity to rise to the occasion.

The details of the " present situation" are in each case different, but the way of meeting it is, in each case, so "accord ing to plan " that the outlines may be sketched to the patient with absolute confidence as soon as the complaint of migraine or of trigeminal neuralgia has been stated, and "organic disease " excluded.

Nevertheless, at different life-periods, the *kinds* of difficulty differ. In the first—that which I have called the pre-sexual life-period—the adjustment that is avoided or is not made is in the context of the home and the school, naturally. In the sexual period of life, the difficulty is in relation to society and to the world: often in the later period—sometimes earlier—the difficulty felt most acutely is one that arises at a higher level of intellectual effort and rationalisation —the kind of difficulty which for some presents itself as a philosophical or ethical, for others as a religious mal-adjustment.

The sex-problem runs like a scarlet thread throughout. There is sex jealousy at home in the pre-sexual period: there is sexual mal-adjustment in the adult period when migraine is most intense and the problem is psychical as well as physical: the same motive may return or continue when physical sexuality is waning, but now as a psychical or ethical problem interfering with the attainment of the calm that is desired.

This is not fanciful; it is obvious enough to anyone who cares to inquire and observe. Perhaps the easiest way to realise how similar are the *life-lines* of all migrainous persons is, in default of clinical experience, to read the lives of the many great men who have been migrainous and who have recorded their physical sufferings. We find, not in their own accounts, but in their biographies, a certain recurrence of phrases and sentences: "a shy sensitive boy"; "much given to brooding"; "unsympathetic parents";

"unhappy early life"; "withdrawal from school"; "struggles"; "vicissitudes"; "imperfect opportunities"; "adverse circumstances"; "marked conscientiousness"; "persistent endeavour"; "repeated failure" and, not unseldom, "ultimate success."

We read, too, that "he never married," or that "his marriage was unhappy." Sometimes the omission of all allusion to domestic life is even more poignant in its suggestiveness than would be mention of infelicity or hint of conjugal dysharmony.

When the patient is a woman the "present state," perhaps even more obviously than when a man is concerned, is one in which *sex-jealousy* is a master-impulse, however carefully concealed. Broadly speaking, all women who are migrainous resent keenly all suggestion of feminine inferiority in general, and feel or would assert their personal superiority to their husbands or to their male associates. The male who is migrainous usually takes the male superiority for granted, but in his inmost heart is humiliated at his failure to impose his own superiority on his womankind.

Now, how does all this come about? We may elucidate the "present position" easily enough; but we want to know how it is that the state of mind leading to the adoption of a definite life-line and course of conduct has been formed.

The beginnings are far back in childhood. Although, often enough, an adult will at first declare, in all good faith, that "the attacks have only come on recently," yet, at subsequent interviews we may be told that it is now remembered how there were like attacks when very young, and, not infrequently, we may be told when the "first attack" took place. The first attack *thus remembered* will *always* be found to be associated with the rise of the inferiority idea in the childish mind, and with its attempted repression. Let me give three or four examples. A professional man, aged 55, recently told me, after several interviews, that his first attack occurred when, as a very small boy, he had been taken for a walk by his father and ridiculed for his inability to answer simple questions in mental arithmetic. And, added, the patient, " I remember, and now see, that afterwards I had headaches when my father asked me to walk with him, because *I then got out of the walks*." Again, a friend of my own recently told me that he distinctly remembers his " first attack " as coming on when, at four or five years of age, an attempt was made to teach him music, and he was ridiculed for stupidity. Ever after the attempt to read music brought on a " sick headache," and so immunity alike from music and from ridicule was secured. In a third case, a little girl of great ability (pushed on one side in favour of less talented brothers) developed headaches when her precocious intelligence was regarded as comical or ridiculous. Now, in adult life, and daily in contact with men whom she controls in business, migraine and neuralgia have been until recently at once her excuses when she failed to impose her will, and her means of retreat when (as often) she feared to fail in imposing her will on male colleagues and subordinates. Her life-line has been the assertion of feminine superiority; she once threw away happiness lest she were dominated by a man, and she formerly found in ill-health her excuse for the life failure she has made through insistence on her own superiority. Like warp and woof, this interplay between the inferiority and superiority ideas can be traced throughout the whole lives of the migrainous.

It is true that many migrainous persons do achieve success: Herschel, du Bois Reymond, Wollaston, Brewer, and many others are in point.

But not all of them succeed in the worldly sense. For, in the migrainous, there is often a curious impulsion to do what they know is "the wrong thing" in the practical conduct of their lives: as if it were their fate, or as if they wished it to be their fate. *They then derive some measure of satisfaction from a demonstration of how well they behave under adverse circumstances, hampered as they are by their own ill-health and the bludgeonings of fate.* They know subconsciously that, in spite of their own ability, they have failed, in perhaps quite ordinary circumstances, and they are, almost to the end, reluctant to acknowledge where and how they have been wrong and have created for themselves the difficulties from which they escape by means of the brain-storms that afford them their excuse. It is, in fact, the consciousness of their own errors in the management of their lives (though unadmitted frankly, even to themselves) that prevents them facing any given situation boldly and that impels them to go on suffering and struggling in "rage and humiliation." If it were otherwise, there would not be the repression of emotional display and the control of self that, turned inwardly, forms the basis of the brain-storm that migraine is, and prevents decisive action in the adjustment of a situation that, however brought about, calls loudly for adjustment.

For there would then be no motive for the restraint : no reason that would appeal to persons of their temperament to suffer silently and in self-deception. The "compulsion" would no longer exist.

Indeed, like most neurotics, the migrainous and the neuralgic, in Adler's words, seek always excuses if life denies the longed-for triumphs, postpone decisions when action is called-for, and "arrange" that what is attained should appear in an intenser light, since gained in spite of suffering. This is as true of the schoolboy with a "bilious attack," as it is of the struggling professional man with an uncongenial wife, and of the intellectually ambitious woman who stifles her sex-impulse.

Moreover, the migrainous and neuralgic are among those who base their actions, as they think, upon reason; they reject intuitional perception. That is why perhaps there is deeper wisdom than may be thought in the notions of those who see in migraine a conflict, or dysharmony, between the cerebro-spinal and the sympathetico-vagal systems!

It will be said: How is all this, even if true, going to help? Well: in the first place, it helps us to understand the patient's life and circumstances, and it guards us against claptrap and easy assurances. It should not lead us to neglect the physical side of the problem; on the contrary, it should help us to understand the *rôle* of the always present organ-inferiority. By treating and adjusting that, as Adler himself said to me recently, we can make the patient "more strong." We can "relieve strain."

But the psychological appreciation enables us to explain to the patient, and to strip him, or help him to strip himself, of his cloak of make-believe. I do not say that this plan can be usefully attempted with children: for them the doctor must appear as the *Deus ex machinâ* who, intervening at the right moment, adjusts the environment to the childish capacity for response, at the same time that he strengthens the child's desire to overcome, and weakens his impulse to "make excuses."

With those of adult life it is otherwise. With them the whole history has to be brought out, sometimes slowly, sometimes more rapidly, so that the patient awakens to a sense of where his real weakness or error has been. The "present" error is sometimes, but not always, of the moral order: more often, I think, it is a failure in practical adjustment to daily life. Often, too, there is some unresolved ethical or intellectual problem. But there is always *some* unacknowledged error in the conduct of life, physical, psychical or spiritual, and the patient must come to realise it himself. This process of realisation may be slow, but sometimes the method that Nathan chose when he spoke to David may be adopted with success. With the elderly, the outlook is at once more and less hopeful than it is with the young and with the adult.

As already said, migraine becomes less consequential with advancing years. The life's work has been done: some practical solution or at least compromise has been attained: the difficulties and fears alike are less keenly felt.

Even, however, when something of the conflict still endures, it is little use stirring up embers that are soon to burn themselves out. Perhaps, too, the old learn otherwise than through the medium of words. Still, even in old age the ruling passion or tendency may remain. One of the most celebrated of migrainous mathematicians and astronomers spent seven or eight of the last years of his long life in abstruse calculations, and then destroyed all evidence of his labour, fearful lest there was initial error, though he himself could not detect or would not admit where, if at all, was the fault.

But for the young adult who has life before him, very much can be done by methods that one must call psychological. I would go so far as to say that even alcohol injections should not be practised in trigeminal neuralgia —though, of course, all sepsis and all " organ-inferiority " must be combated—unless a psychological solution s first attempted. Otherwise, what we do may be no more rational than would be the amputation of the paralysed and anæsthetic limb of an hysterical girl.

Only the merest outline of the " treatment " necessary can here be given. The physician, sure of his ground, must first establish the " present difficulty " that obtains in every case. Then he may gather the details of the life history, and may point out to the patient how the " life-line " has been constant, how the same attitude has been always maintained in face of apparent difficulties in the different spheres and relations of activity. He may, and often will, be successful in bringing to the conscious mind recollections of the earliest difficulties experienced and of the manner in which they were met. He must endeavour to allow conviction to come to the patient rather than to enforce it on him: but he may lead him to see that it is persistence in the life-line, so long ago laid out, that is leading to the present failure to adjust a difficult situation, to the "rage and humiliation" that is suffered but suppressed, and to the physical demonstration of the mental suffering. He probably may, and certainly will if he adopts a didactic *rôle*, meet with obstinacy and unwillingness to admit anything but action dictated by the best and highest motives. But, if the patient himself sees where the initial error has been, half the battle has been won. Then comes the question of the adjustment of the present difficulty, the settlement of the urgent problem. If the physician *dictates* a solution, nothing is gained. The patient—to use the language of the revivalist—once "convicted" must "work out his own salvation."

And here, help can be given. The patient can be brought to see that the conflict may and will be solved if and when the practical problem is removed from its apparent context to a higher or wider one. Thus, what appears to be a personal difficulty, to be decided on personal grounds from personal motives, can be shown easy of solution when approached from the point of view of the claims of society.

Instinct may demand flight from danger in battle, and ingenious personal reasons may be alleged to approve such flight. But the appeal to the interests of the unit of which the individual is but a part, may bring a more satisfactory decision. So, too, in the intellectual or ethical sphere.

A problem that may appear insoluble in science will lose its difficulty when brought into relation with metaphysics, and what is a riddle in metaphysics is answered by the highest philosophy of all.

After all, this is only the method of

Science itself. Newton solved the problem of the falling apple when he raised the question to the level of the solar system, and, in doing so, he solved, for the time being, the problem of that system.

Moreover, the same method was urged, so many years ago, by Plotinus, for the healing of disorders bodily and mental, as well as spiritual.

Plotinus, the Neo-Platonist, held that the disorders of the body depend upon improper direction by the "soul" —or unconscious mind: those of the "soul" upon the state of the "nous" —or conscious mind; and those of the "nous" upon estrangement from the One. Hence, cure of bodily disorder must depend upon adjustment of the unconscious mind, and that again upon the "nous," as the clarity of the "nous" upon its still higher relations.

The same idea and the same method has been expressed in many languages, at many centres of culture, and by many religious and medical systems. We should not be afraid to meet it, and to make use of it: nor should we shrink from pursuing it to its logical conclusion. In many, very many, of the disorders that we have to treat, the urgency for the application of physical methods is, and must be, undisputed. Yet the change that may attend the successful exploration of the minds of those who suffer from migraine and neuralgia is so remarkable, so profound, and so lasting, that one is tempted to use the phrase spoken by revivalists and philosophers alike, and to say that it is indeed a process of "conversion" or of "reconciliation." We may, if we like, with Wittgenstein, think of Kant's left-handed glove turned round in four-dimensional space, so becoming right-handed. Or we may suppose, in the language of physiologists, that the endocrine balance has been restored, and the sympathetic and cerebro-spinal systems have been reconciled. But the facts are as I have stated them, and may be easily verified.

* * * *

The Christian Scientists, amongst

others, seem sometimes to see farther than do the purely "organicist" physicians. On the other hand, the Freudians miss something, as in another direction do perhaps the followers o Jung. Silberer perhaps leaned too far towards mysticism of a wrong kind.

But Adler, in his recognition of the relation between organ-inferiorities and the part played by psychoses, and in his insistence on the superiority-aim, has made a very great advance. Only, if I may say so, he seems in error in reducing the conflict that is in the mind of every neurotic to one between an *innate* superiority-aim, and an inferiority-sense implanted *by circumstances.* In so doing, he maintains the patient's idea that he or she is the victim of injustice. Now, call it what we will, there is in each one of us an *instinct* opposed to what is variously called the Superiority-aim, the Pleasure-principle, or the Libido. So much has recently been recognised by Freud himself, in his last book *Beyond the Pleasure-principle.* But did not the author of the *Analogy of Religion* grasp what is at issue when he declared the "Authorities in the Polity of the Soul" to be two: Conscience and Self-Love? It does not seem to me that there is any real difference between Freud's Pleasure-principle, Jung's Libido, Adler's Superiority-aim, and Butler's Self-Love, save perhaps this, that the term self-love is the most comprehensive and includes definitely the conservation-instinct. On the other hand, Freud's new innate principle seems to me but an imperfect *alias* for Butler's Conscience. By conscience I do not mean merely the admission of moral turpitude in respect of particular acts, but something innate and more general, and which may be described as an inferiority-sense, not in respect of our fellows and rivals, but in respect of some higher standard which we should recognise.

And perhaps, when we talk as we now do so much about the conscious, the unconscious, and the subconscious, we are really "repressing" recognition of what Butler called the Conscience, and of what Otto, in his *Idea of the Holy*, calls the Numinous.

We may fitly remember in this connection how, at the end, Kant declared two things to fill him with wonder and amazement: the moral law within and the starry sky above him. And there is a close parallel between the migraine of the school-child whose self-love is wounded by the failure he resents, and that of the astronomer who does not willingly admit his failure to comprehend, by force of intellect alone, the riddle of the Universe.

* * *

In each and every migrainous, and in most violent neuralgics, there is repression of the "rage and humiliation" felt in face of some problem —practical, ethical, or intellectual— that appears insoluble. The problem remains insoluble so long as personal responsibility for the failure in action, or the personal inadequacy for the failure in thought, remains unacknowledged; and so long as the decision which must follow the admission is thereby avoided.

The brain-storm of the migrainous, and that of the neuralgic, are defence and flight and excuse mechanisms, analogous to those which, during the War, we found exhibited in face of physical danger.

The peculiar characters of the paroxysms are in each case determined by the organ-inferiority or state present. In the one it is an affection, or imperfection of the optic tracts, from cornea to thalamus and cortex, that may be expressed as revealed by lack of perfect correspondence between the two sides: in the other, it is a state or inferiority affecting the whole domain of the fifth nerve on one side, from periphery to Gasserian ganglion, and higher still, sometimes. In each case the inferiority, lack of balance, or pathological condition becomes manifest or potent under stress that may be physical, psychical or intellectual, in the main, but which is usually as complex as is the apparent relation of mind and body, of organ states and emotion-states, of intellectual and cerebral activity.